REFLECTIONS:
NURSES AS
EDUCATORS

REFLECTIONS: NURSES AS EDUCATORS

B. A. Nurse Educator

iUniverse, Inc.
New York Bloomington Shanghai

REFLECTIONS: NURSES AS EDUCATORS

iUniverse books may be ordered through booksellers or by contacting:

iUniverse
1663 Liberty Drive
Bloomington, IN 47403
www.iuniverse.com
1-800-Authors (1-800-288-4677)

Because of the dynamic nature of the Internet, any Web addresses or links contained in this book may have changed since publication and may no longer be valid.

ISBN: 978-0-595-44781-7 (pbk)
ISBN: 978-0-595-89099-6 (ebk)

Printed in the United States of America

FOR ALL THE NURSE EDUCATORS
OF TOMORROW

The School of Nursing at George Mason University
wishes to gratefully acknowledge
Epsilon Zeta Chapter of Sigma Theta Tau International
for its generous funding of this project.

Contents

Contributors xi

Preface xv

Moving from Clinician to Preceptor/Nurse Educator Role 1

Self-Reflection 3
Kathy Green

Reality Shock 5
Megan M. Davis

What Do We Owe Our Students? 7
Adele McGowan

Lifelong Learner 9
Nagaina Simmons

Many Times a Novice 13
Carol Gavin

I Can Do It All 15
Pamela Juliet John

The Joy of Teaching 17
Shirley Pearson

Making a Difference 21

Making a Difference as a Nurse Educator 23
Alisa Olson

My Hero 25
Marian Harmon

Room to Grow 28
Shirley Pearson

Asking Questions 31
Paige Migliozzi

GI "Jane" as Patient Advocate 33
Hettie C. Mercer

A Defining Moment 35
Karen Livornese

Making a Difference in a Life 38
Nadia Ali

Little "Feats" of Wonder 40
Nagaina Simmons

Making a Difference in a Journey 43
Fleur D. May

Mentoring Clinical Nurse Educators of the Future 45

Even Teachers Need A Little Guidance Now and Then. 47
Amy O'Neill

A Thousand Little Steps. 51
Karen Backo

Each Individual is Unique 53
Deirdre Dorsey

Positive Attitude 55
Emily Sperlazza

Wanted: Mentors! 57
Comfort Avovabey

A Love of Nursing and a Passion to Teach. 59
Megan M. Davis

Mentoring to Uncover Possibilities 60
Sarah Mossburg

Meeting the Challenges of Nursing Education. 61
Shirley Pearson

Contributors

Nadia Ali, BSN, RN graduated in 1993 from the Aga Khan University, Karachi, Pakistan. She will obtain her MSN in Summer 2008 from George Mason with a focus on nursing education. She currently works as a staff nurse in the Telemetry Unit at Inova Fair Oaks Hospital.

Comfort Avovabey, MSN, RN received a Diploma in Nursing and baccalaureate degree from the University of Ghana, graduating in 1991 and 1994 respectively. She obtained a MSN in May 2008 from George Mason with a focus on nursing education and currently works as a staff nurse in OB/L&D setting. She has also taught as adjunct faculty at George Mason.

Karen Backo, MSN, RNC received her BSN from Loma Linda University and her MSN in Nursing Education from George Mason. Karen holds a post-baccalaureate certificate in Perfusion Science from The Johns Hopkins Hospital School of Perfusion Science and has been certified by the American Board of Cardiovascular Perfusion. For the past six years, her practice has been as a staff nurse, RN IV in the Family Birthing Center at Fauquier Hospital and is NCC certified in both Inpatient Obstetric and Maternal Newborn Nursing. She is also a Certified Legal Nurse Consultant. Karen is currently an Adjunct Faculty member at George Mason teaching maternal-infant health in the clinical setting.

Pamela Cangelosi, PhD, RN, CNE is an Associate Professor in the School of Nursing at George Mason. Her doctoral work focused on education with an emphasis on RN to BSN education. She is currently the Coordinator of George Mason's graduate Nurse Educator track and doing research related to accelerated baccalaureate second degree nursing education and the transition of clinical nurses to clinical educators.

Megan Murphy Davis, PhD, RN has practiced nursing since 1976. Her areas of interest include OB/GYN and pediatrics. Megan has taught undergraduate and graduate nursing students and is currently the school nurse for a 1,200 student middle school in Loudoun County, Virginia.

Deirdre Dorsey, MSN, RN worked as a Public Health Nurse II at Fairfax County Health Department, Virginia, while pursuing her graduate degree with a focus on nursing education at George Mason University.

Sharon Favazza, MSN, RN has used her nursing skills and education to support the health and well being of indigenous people living in Southeast Asia for the past fourteen years. Passionate about improving their standards of health care, Sharon is commonly seen conducting medical clinics in remote villages. Sharon believes life-long learning is the basis for quality nursing practice and will begin her studies for a doctoral degree in nursing this fall.

Suzy Tacaraya Fehr, MS, RN, CNA-BC has a passion for nursing informatics and currently works at Inova Alexandria Hospital while completing her doctoral dissertation on *Nurses' Perceptions of Using Handheld Technologies at the Bedside*.

Carol Gavin, MSN, RNC works at Inova Fair Oaks in case management. She has been a nurse over 30 years, specializing in psychiatric and mental health nursing for the past 15 years. She obtained a MSN at George Mason in nursing education in May 2008.

Kathy Green, BS, RN has been a nurse for sixteen years. She is currently working as a clinical nursing supervisor at Prince William Hospital in Manassas, Virginia. She will graduate from George Mason in 2008 with a MSN in nursing education.

Marian Harmon, MSN, RN has been a public health nurse in School Health with Arlington County DHS since 1997. She is currently working as a public health nurse supervisor in School Health. Her previous nursing experience includes NICU, postpartum and lactation consulting. Marian received her BSN in 1980 and MSN in May 2008, both from George Mason. Her graduate studies focused on nursing education.

Kathy Howey has been a clinical nurse for 28 years. She received an AD in Nursing from Shenandoah College in 1980 and a MSN and Certificate in Nursing Education from George Mason University in 2007 and 2008, respectively. She is currently working in Labor & Delivery at Reston Hospital Center and as adjunct faculty for George Mason University, teaching Maternal-Newborn Nursing in the clinical setting. She is proud to be a contributor to this book and hopes it will inspire other clinical nurses to consider a career in nursing education.

Elizabeth Itote, MSN, CNM earned a Certificate in Nursing Education from George Mason and works in physicians and midwives collaborative practice in Alexandria, Virginia.

Pamela John worked in a Mission Hospital in India as a Clinical Nursing Instructor for five years and in New York City as a Case Manager with the United Cerebral Palsy Association. She currently works on the Medical/Oncology Unit at INOVA Fair Oaks Hospital.

Karen Livornese, MA, RN received a BSN from the University of Rochester and is an ANCC Board Certified Mental Health Nurse. She currently serves as an ACRP Certified Clinical Research Nurse Coordinator for the Gynecologic Disease Center at Walter Reed Army Medical Center. Karen also holds a BA from Georgetown University, an MA from Virginia Tech, and is currently pursuing a MSN in nursing administration at George Mason University.

Fleur May, RN received her undergraduate degree in Nursing from George Mason University. She is currently a NICU nurse and a graduate student at George Mason completing her MSN in nursing education.

Adele McGowan, BSN, RNC has worked for over 20 years in the Neonatal Intensive Care Unit at the Inova Fairfax Hospital for Children. She currently works as the New Hire Support Coordinator for the NICU while pursuing her MSN degree from George Mason.

Hettie Mercer, MSN, RN, CGRN spent fifteen years as the charge nurse for Sibley Memorial Hospital's Endoscopy Unit. She currently is the Nurse Manager of the Outpatient Procedure Suite at Sibley Memorial Hospital.

Paige Migliozzi, RN works as a Clinical Instructor in the Inova Learning Network at Inova Fairfax Hospital. She received a BS from Virginia Tech, a BSN at George Mason and will receive a MSN from George Mason in December 2008.

Sarah Mossburg, RN has a BSN from the University of Pennsylvania and a Masters degree in Health Systems Administration from Georgetown University. Her current position is the Director of Professional Practice and Magnet Program Director at Mount Vernon Hospital. She is responsible for hospital-wide issues related to nursing professional practice, specifically issues related to nursing quality, education, and research. Sarah is also the site coordinator for the National Database of Nursing Quality Indicators (NDNQI).

Alisa Olson, MSN, RN has been a critical care nurse for 15 years. She graduated from Montgomery College in 1993 and later received her BSN from the University of Delaware. Alisa works as a clinical manager in a 14 bed SICU at the Washington Hospital Center in Washington, D.C. She received her MSN in May 2008 from George Mason and has accepted a position as adjunct faculty at Georgetown University.

Amy O'Neill, RN worked at INOVA Fairfax Hospital on the Labor, Delivery, and Recovery unit while earning her MSN in nursing education at George Mason University.

Shirley Pearson, MSN, RN has practiced nursing for 24 years in a variety of clinical areas including ICU, PACU, Home Health, and currently the ED. She has wide experience in adjunct faculty, preceptor, and staff development educator roles while striving to define nursing as the art of caring.

Nagaina Simmons, RN has been a staff nurse, Clinician IV, at Virginia Hospital Center for approximately six years, working in the Neonatal Intensive Care Unit. She graduated from the University of Virginia with a BSN and went straight into her clinical specialty. She is currently a graduate student at George Mason, pursuing a MSN in nursing education, and hopes to graduate in May 2009.

Jeanne Sorrell, PhD, RN is a Professor in the School of Nursing at George Mason University. Her doctoral work focused on curriculum and instruction and writing. She is currently teaching in George Mason's Nurse Educator track and doing research in *Ethics of Respect for Spirituality in Persons Living with Alzheimer's Disease.*

Emily Sperlazza, RN received an Associate Degree in Nursing from Germanna Community College, BA in Psychology from Mary Washington College, and plans to receive a MSN in Nursing from George Mason University in August 2008. Her clinical background is in Obstetrics/Labor & Delivery, hospice, and community nursing. She currently works as adjunct nursing faculty at Germanna Community College and as a PRN Hospice nurse. She finds nursing education fascinating!

Preface

This book grew out of a new venture in the School of Nursing at George Mason University that focused on preparation of Clinical Nurse Educators. In May 2007, participants in the Clinical Nurse Educator Academy wrote stories about their experiences in moving from roles as experienced clinicians into new roles as clinical preceptors and educators, where they often felt like novices. We found these stories so meaningful that we proposed to our class of Nurse Educator graduate students in Spring 2008 that we implement a collaborative project to publish the stories in a book that could be enjoyed by other nurses, especially those moving into a new role of Clinical Nurse Educator.

The students immediately became excited about the project and worked closely to gather stories that would convey important aspects of the role of nurses as clinical preceptors and clinical nurse educators. The result is *Reflections: Nurses as Educators*, in which the students reflect on their own experiences as nurses and nurse educators. There are stories of *Moving from Clinician to Preceptor/Nurse Educator Role*, *Making a Difference*, and *Mentoring Clinical Nurse Educators of the Future*. Each story reflects events that made important differences in the career of the nurse authors as they moved toward new roles as preceptors or clinical nurse educators.

With the current shortage of nurse educators, we hope this book will help to convey the wonderful possibilities for careers in nursing education, especially clinical nurse education. Proceeds from the sale of the book will be used for projects to benefit nursing students and faculty involved in clinical nursing education. We applaud the work and commitment of the students who have produced this book and hope you enjoy it!

Jeanne Sorrell and Pamela Cangelosi

Moving from Clinician to Preceptor/Nurse Educator Role

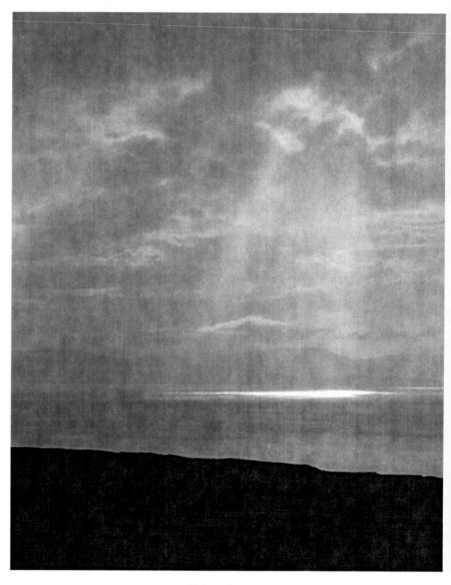

Light on Water 2
by Tony Hisgett

Self-Reflection
Kathy Green

Change is good and necessary. It has been my experience, however, that with any change, there are growing pains. People tend to get complacent with the status quo and rebel against anything that resembles change. Changing roles from an expert clinician to a novice nurse educator definitely causes me to self-reflect. I have many concerns. Will I have all the right answers? Will I understand all of the students' questions? Will I be a positive role model? Will I be approachable? Will I communicate clearly? These are just a few of the questions that I ask myself.

I think about all of the instructors I had during my clinical experience. None were perfect. I am not sure there is such a thing, yet I learned from all of them. Each instructor had valuable information to share. I was eager for the knowledge. I watched and absorbed every little detail.

There was only one instructor who left a negative imprint in my memory. I will never forget her. She was extremely critical of all of the students and made us feel inferior. She would yell and belittle us in front of the other students. It is because of her that I try to be intensely aware of my own words and body language when I am interacting with my coworkers and patients. As a nursing supervisor, I am in a position of authority. I could easily make my nursing staff feel uncomfortable. That is not the environment, however, in which I want to work. I firmly believe that all people need to feel respected and valued. By nurturing and building up my nurses, I find that they are happier and more productive. This attitude is then conveyed to the patients.

I think about my core values of respect and nurturing others when I question how I will be as a nurse educator. Even though there will be a transition period, I think that all of the qualities that make me a successful nursing supervisor will help me to be a successful nurse educator.

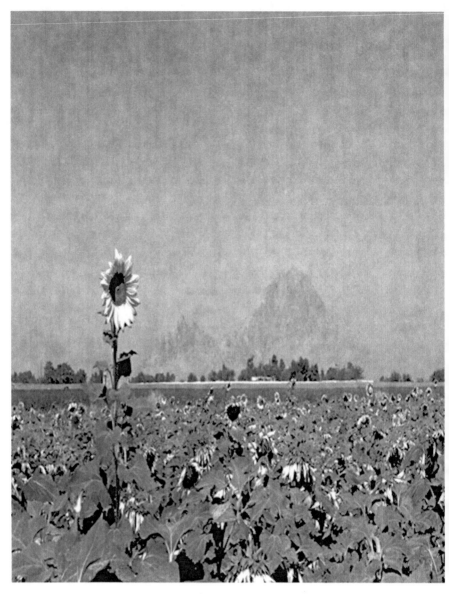

I Shall Fight to Stay Alive
by Hamed Saber

Reality Shock
Megan M. Davis

This past school year I reentered the work force after nearly a decade "off". I had been busy these past nine years fighting breast cancer, raising my young children, and then nursing my elderly parents. I came back to work for myself. You see, I missed being what I am at my core: I am a nurse.

While "unemployed" I enjoyed years of volunteer work—running a Girl Scout camp, being the "Band Mom", and serving on two schools PTAs. Now I was returning to my nursing career and I decided to start back as a middle school nurse. The position was attractive because the school was close to my home and matched my younger children's schedules. I knew many of the students and their mothers from Scouts, so how difficult could this be? The answer in a word: Very!

I am a well prepared nurse. I worked as a nurse for many years in a variety of settings and capacities. I hold several degrees and love research. I have taught nurses. I was not prepared, however, for the reality shock of being a novice after all these years. School nursing turned out to be far different than I had ever imagined. In orientation, I was told that the cliché description of school nursing, "Band-Aids and Bufferin," was not reality. Boy, was that the truth! School nursing involves a mastery of ever-changing immunization requirements, vision and hearing screenings, medication administration, sports injuries, medical illnesses, simple first aid, emergency skills, and the daily work of keeping students in class. This work requires a large dose of psychiatry of children, their families, and school staff. I found myself a student again for the first time in years. I reviewed pediatrics and read school nursing texts, emergency texts, and CDC reports. But I longed for a mentor.

School budgets are tight and teacher-focused. Nurses are considered auxiliary staff. Indeed, in some school systems there are no nurses. My nursing department is stretched very thin. Orientation was short and jammed full of information. A six-inch thick nursing manual was presented in class. Talk about sensory overload! The computer system was down the day I was to be taught how to use it. "No worries!" I was told. Each school has several secretaries to help. My secretaries, however, were all new. After the first month, the only secretary with any medical background (she was an EMT) resigned. Yes, I could call nurses at other schools but the sense of isolation was undeniable. My school with 1,200 students and 150 staff was in my hands, alone.

Interestingly, another school nurse from my county was a graduate student at George Mason. She asked for feedback about our orientation experience for a paper she was writing. For the past 12 years she worked for our county as a school nurse. She wanted a fresh perspective of what it was like to be a "novice." Our responses were promised to be kept confidential. Only two of us responded from our orientation group of 12. How disappointing!

Now the school year is nearly over. I appreciate the chance to be a nurse again after a "professional" break. I appreciate working with patients, but I miss the fellowship of nurses. The lack of a mentor made the job far more difficult than it had to be. I have made myself a mental note that when I return to teaching, I will remember how it felt to be a novice. Being a novice is a good thing. It means you are growing and learning new things. But now I realize one thing more—every novice, regardless of previous areas of expertise, needs a mentor.

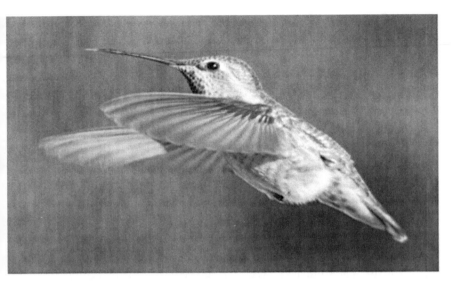

Anna's Hummingbird
by Noel Zia Lee

What Do We Owe Our Students?

Adele McGowan

Advancing in my clinical nursing career was a process that was gradual, unassuming, and rather comfortable. I worked as a newly graduated nurse in medical-surgical nursing (because that's what one usually did in the '70s), and then switched to a specialty area. Over a span of 28 years, I became increasingly competent and proficient in the pediatric and newborn arena. I climbed the clinical ladder as far as I could go. I became certified in my field and was considered somewhat of an expert. With ever-increasing knowledge, experience, and confidence, I felt accomplished, credible, and well respected. All was right with the world! Why would I upset this perfectly stocked apple cart? Because another opportunity became available and I decided to leave my comfort zone and forge ahead. This was a scary proposition for me, however, because this particular opportunity would not help me advance at the bedside and did not follow the natural progression of my career path. Woe is me!

My new (and current) job is being the New Hire Coordinator for a Neonatal Intensive Care Unit (NICU). As the person responsible for most "New Hire" issues, I thought that I had a fairly good grasp of what the job entailed and how I could expand the role to encompass both new *and* "old" hire support, student placements, recruitment initiatives, and still work that occasional shift at the bed-side. I was pumped and excited to get those new nurses assigned to good precep-tors, to orient students to the NICU, and to do the best that I could in this new role. Although I was definitely a beginner in this new role when I started almost four years ago, and received only minimal orientation, I was not too apprehensive and felt that if I came upon an unfamiliar situation, I could probably "just wing it". I had a positive attitude, good intentions, and support from management. Plus, it meant a pay raise and no holiday/week-end requirements! This might just work out fine. And then I had my "ah, ha" moment …

Shortly after starting this new position, I took a trip to California and brought along some nursing journals to read on the plane. I don't remember which partic-ular state we were flying over at the time, but I do remember that I was in the plane when I read something that really gave me a jolt. It was an article about clinical experiences for nursing students and the responsibilities of both student *and* instructor. The student is owed (and deserves) an instructor, preceptor, and/or unit facilitator who is well versed and properly educated on evidence-based methods regarding knowledge acquisition, effective teaching strategies, and sup-portive relationship building. The new and "old" hires merit someone who understands how psychomotor and social skills are acquired and enhanced and where each person is on his/her career journey. Good intentions can only go so far.

I knew then that although I had many years of life and career experience, I was a mere "babe" in the area of staff and student development. I also realized that I must further my formal education and keep current on issues related to this new endeavor because that is what is owed to those whom I support and orient. Hopefully, I have become increasingly competent, proficient, and credible in this new role. I don't think, however, that I ever will (or should) become too comfort-able in this position. There is too much at stake for that to happen.

Lifelong Learner
Nagaina Simmons

Moving from "expert" to "novice" involves change, a kind of starting over. As with any new undertaking or role, there is a sense of apprehension and a moment where one questions his or her ability to learn new information and accomplish new tasks. I recall feeling this way as a new graduate. I remember thinking: I went to one of the best schools in the state, so I should have learned all I needed to know ... right? I even passed my NCLEX exam the first time, so I must be adequately prepared as nurse ... don't you think? But as I started my new career as a nursery/NICU/delivery room nurse, I realized that there was *a lot* I did not know. I had only one pediatric rotation, although I had the opportunity to do my practicum in a pediatric clinic. So I guess I felt comfortable with one thing: *giving injections.* The rest of it was news to me.

I must admit, that this was very unsettling for me. I'm the kind of person who likes to know everything upfront before I do it. I thoroughly researched what kind of car I should buy, what kind of life insurance is best, what the difference is between a 401(k) and an IRA—you know, those kinds of things. But when it came to resuscitating a newborn, starting an IV in tiny veins, or caring for 28-week twins, I felt like a nursing student all over again. Thank goodness the nurses on my unit didn't "eat their young". I was fortunate enough to have two good preceptors during my orientation. They were patient, kind, understanding, yet firm. That was exactly what I needed. I definitely wouldn't say I was an expert by the end of orientation, but these nurses did lay a good foundation for me to one day acquire that status (which of course, after only five years as a nurse, I have yet to reach).

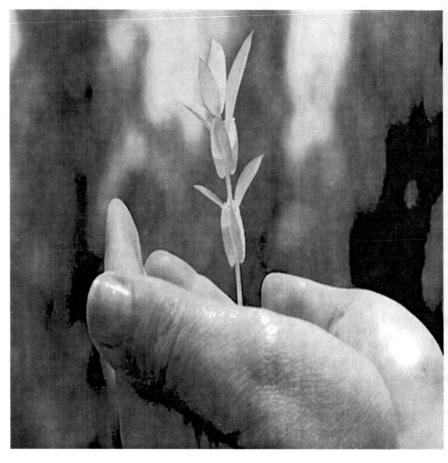

Grow Trees
by Thiru Murugan

I also remember having this "unsettling" feeling the very first time I had to precept a new nurse. Granted, I was becoming more and more comfortable caring for my patients and gaining more and more knowledge of my specialty. I also liked teaching the newer nurses on the unit and serving as a resource. But was I ready to take new graduates under my wing and teach them to be NICU nurses? I recall not knowing where to begin. One specific preceptee was an older nurse, had three kids, and had experience as an Emergency Medical Technician. I began to ask myself: Would it be awkward because of our age difference? Do I begin with the basics or start at a higher level? What if she asks me a question I don't know? Am I really ready for this? I dealt with all these questions (and more!) throughout "our" orientation. With a few bumps along the way, we both got through it. We developed a great relationship and to this day she still works on the unit; she serves as charge nurse and continues to show great enthusiasm for what she does. I guess I didn't do *that* bad!

When I think about what it will be like to be a nurse educator, these are the incidents that come to mind. I remember feeling unsettled, unsure, apprehensive, and mildly excited with each of these new endeavors. I love teaching and I know that being a nurse educator is something I've been called to do. I know that if I am kind, patient, understanding, yet firm, just like my preceptors were, my students will gain a lot from me as their teacher. I'm sure all of these feelings will resurface again once I start my academic career. The trick is to remember those times when I was a novice. Hard work, patience, and passion will help me to one day obtain that expertise I once felt I had. But I must admit that, as I have matured in this profession, sometimes I like being a novice: it means there is so much more knowledge out there for me to obtain. And if we think about it, you really can't be an expert and be an educator. Learning is continuous and it is life-long. That's what I love about education. I aspire to not only be an educator, but a lifelong learner as well.

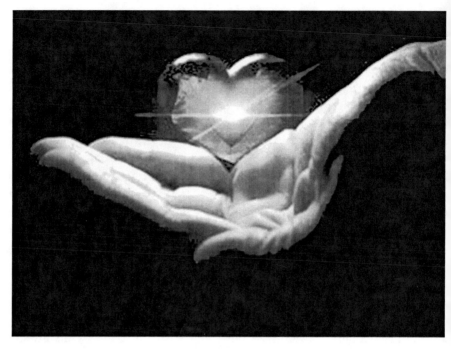

Heart In Hand
Anonymous

Many Times a Novice
Carol Gavin

I have been a nurse for 32 years. I have been a novice many times. I have been an expert a few times. For me, one of the best things about nursing is the variety of work that is offered as a nurse. I had been a medical-surgical nurse for 15 years when I took a new job as a psychiatric nurse on weekend nights, (a great job when I had young children). When I think back on that novice role, I have good memories. I plan to use what helped me in the past as a novice. I was enthusiastic and wanted to learn as much as I could from the people around me. I asked questions at the right time and really listened. I shared my delight when I "got" something and I know it made my coworkers feel good about the knowledge they had, but sometimes took for granted. Being a novice makes me feel young. By the time I left this particular hospital, five years later, I had become a supervisor, managing and solving problems for the whole 55-bed hospital. I had a similar experience when I became a novice manager in a community hospital. My director mentored me and I was enthusiastic and committed to becoming a good manager.

There have been more examples in my career of where I have made a choice to be a novice. I allow myself to be a novice, to not know everything and to learn from others and the job itself. My experience has been that if it is a good fit, I am eventually able to become an expert at the job. I have confidence in myself and I have developed the confidence by taking risks to do something new.

So I am very excited to be a new teacher. I love nursing and I want to help new nurses enjoy all that nursing can give to us. I want new nurses to know it is OK not to know everything. I want them to see that the most valuable thing we give our patients is a part of ourselves, to care, and to be with that person for that time to let them know they are not alone.

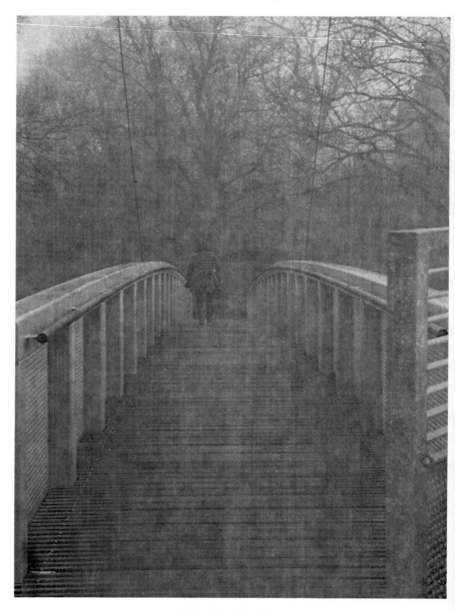

Bridge Over River Soar
by Chris Hoare

I Can Do It All
Pamela Juliet John

A nurse can never forget her beginning days as a new graduate, no matter what great heights she reaches in her career. Some nurses opt to work in small settings like doctors' offices as soon as they graduate after they hear "scary" stories from their friends or acquaintances who had bitter experiences during their orientation period. I know some new graduates who went into different fields like marketing and real estate in order to feel "safe". On a brighter note, there are many students who graduate with a great desire and enthusiasm to help their patients. Hopefully, they also get paired up with some good "sensitive" preceptors who make their learning process smooth and easy.

After I graduated, I had the opportunity to work in a Mission Hospital. Being a charitable institution, the hospital did not have a big teaching faculty. Hence, I worked as a Clinical Instructor teaching the students and helped out in the learning lab. I worked harder as an educator than as a student! I spent most of my time in the lab and hospital with the students. Honestly, most of the time I was constantly anxious, wondering if I did things right. At least I didn't hear much criticism. People were kind. Maybe because I already participated in the teaching and orientation process fresh out of nursing school, transitioning was not a very difficult process. My preceptor was very helpful.

Now working as a Clinician/Charge Nurse in an acute setting, I had the experience of precepting two nurses—one who moved from a long term care setting and another extern. Being on a really hectic medical floor with a whole pod of patients, it felt a bit difficult to take time to orient and teach. It slowed down my tasks for the day and sometimes I think I was not very "pleasant", though I could justify my "not very pleasant attitude" to myself.

I still remember an incident while I was precepting. I had to change a Vac dressing and I was already running late. The patient was waiting anxiously. I was looking for the new nurse so that I could take her with me to show her the dressing change, as she had never seen a Vac dressing before. Even though she knew that we had planned this earlier, she was in another patient's room chatting with the relative. Meanwhile, the patient got upset with me, saying that I forgot her dressing. At that moment I decided that I was never going to show my preceptee anything unless she stayed with me and showed readiness to learn. Though I didn't say anything outwardly, she could sense that I was not very pleased. Later, I heard that the relative was very sick and wanted to talk to somebody. I felt terrible that I didn't even take time to talk to this nurse about what happened (I did show her how to do a Vac dressing though!).

The Clinical Nurse Educator Academy at George Mason was an eye opener for me. I couldn't help but recollect the pressure during my days as a preceptor. I did my best and the evidence is that both of the nurses who I precepted are still in nursing. I still keep in touch with them. I wonder, though, how much of a role model I was! I haven't volunteered to be a preceptor lately. I am sure my approach as a preceptor will definitely be different the next time when I have a new graduate working with me. I want to be a good, sensitive preceptor/educator able to recognize the needs of a new graduate/student, be supportive throughout the orientation period, and at the same time not overwhelm the orientee with too much information.

Being a novice myself in the role of a preceptor, I don't think I was very positive in terms of "positive feedback and constructive criticism". I would really want the new graduates and new nurses to have great memories of their orientation period. A good beginning will be an encouraging factor to help new graduates stay in nursing and easily adapt to new roles as clinicians, educators, and nursing leaders. I am looking forward to serving as a guide, supporter, and a stimulator in whatever nursing position I pursue.

The Joy of Teaching
Shirley Pearson

Nursing is a wonderful profession to be a part of. Each encounter with patients and their families is its own unique experience. Every day nurses touch someone's life in a different way. Nurses don't have to be experts in the profession to provide and promote care to others. We all began as novices and continue to grow with experience and education.

Nursing is very versatile in that you can experience all different types of nursing. I have changed nursing areas seven times to experience more of what nursing has to offer. I guess I've been a novice many times throughout my career. Each time, however, has been a little different. Surprisingly, I have never felt the novice role in the way I did when I graduated from nursing school. I brought different skill sets to each new setting. One of the biggest changes and challenges has been from an office role back to a fast-paced acute care setting.

In the past, I enjoyed the role of clinical nurse educator. There were several reasons for pursuing other roles in nursing. Two of these reasons were student attitudes and lack of facility support.

Years ago, I worked in the acute care setting as a Staff Development Instructor. Each fall and spring I provided clinical instruction to second year nursing students. The community college provided a set of books and clinical objectives, as well as a list of the nursing skills the students were expected to learn. The nursing faculty would call occasionally during the clinical rotation to check on things. As the years rolled by, I began to notice that the students enrolled in the program were there because nursing salaries were more competitive and jobs were available. What I didn't see was the caring attitude of wanting to make a difference in the profession. It was disheartening. I noticed a lack of enthusiasm in learning and participating in clinical lessons. The thoughts and attitudes of these future nurses were concerning to me because they fell short of my expectations. At the time, I didn't know what or how to provide these students with guidance and mentoring for their development as nurses.

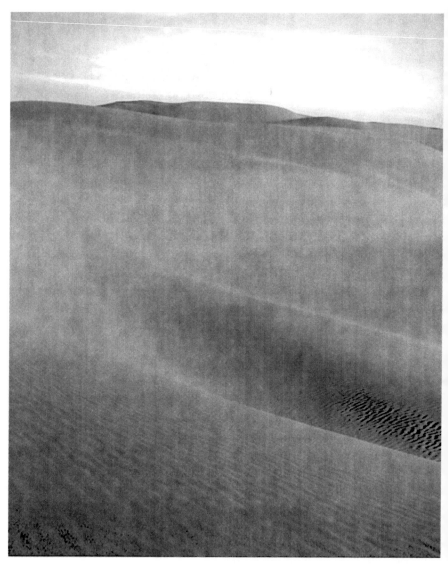

Erthreality of Eternity
by Hamed Saber

Initially, I was blinded by my own enthusiasm of wanting to provide these students with excellent clinical experience and at the same time provide my employer (the acute care facility) with quality work. Each clinical rotation I had double the amount of work. My employer expected the same job to be done whether there were students involved or not. Plus my own expectation of "I can do it all" came in conflict with a work-life balance: I couldn't burn the candle at both ends for long without getting burned myself. After six years, I chose to leave the job before I became one of those instructors who did not like their profession, making themselves and those around them miserable.

Several years after leaving this job, I realized how much I did enjoy teaching nursing students. I felt the need for more education to provide a theoretical basis and learning opportunities to help me on my journey. I also realized the importance of having current knowledge of what's happening in the real world of acute care nursing. I want to provide current stories in my teaching, so I accepted a nursing position in an acute care facility to fulfill that need. Being a novice again brought back old memories. I began my job there shortly before eight new graduate nurses. I quickly realized I was mentoring these new nurses in their transition from student to nurse.

I had concerns about these nurses entering a specialty area without having basic nursing practice. These nurses were given approximately six months of orientation, which consisted of little classroom theory. The new graduates were then placed with a mentor who may have been at the hospital one or more years. Many concerns raced through my head, including safety of the patients, safety for the staff, and legal issues, including medication administration. My concerns were whether we were going to give these nurses the time and experiences they needed to grow in the fast-paced unit where everything seemed like an emergency. I thought: How am I going to bridge these new graduates into functioning as competent nurses?

At the time, I was not a preceptor because I was quite new myself, but I felt responsible for these nurses. I wanted them to have a positive experience and stay engaged in nursing. There are so many things to ponder such as providing the new graduate nurses with evidence-based practice, fostering time management skills, and being a professional role model. Promoting trust in these new graduate nurses is also difficult. Sometimes it's difficult to know when to step in so they learn skills and not flounder, always thinking about safety for both the patient and the nurse. Preceptors often work with a full patient load and provide instruction to new grads as well. This may deter others from seeking to fulfill this role as preceptor due to the heavy work load. With budgetary constraints and decreased staff, administrators seem to expect more with less—a nurse preceptor working with a nurse on orientation adds up to two nurses to cover the patients. It's that double-edged sword. You have both jobs that need to be done. You strive to do what you can to keep the new staff on the job and not become fed up with lack of support and the heavy work load.

I still struggle with acting as a preceptor for a new nurse in an area of practice that I have had little experience with myself. I can provide new staff with basic nursing concepts and safety in caring for many patients, but I too am trying to become competent in this new arena. I hardly feel like an expert, but with each day, I gain valuable experience that I can share with a novice.

Making a Difference

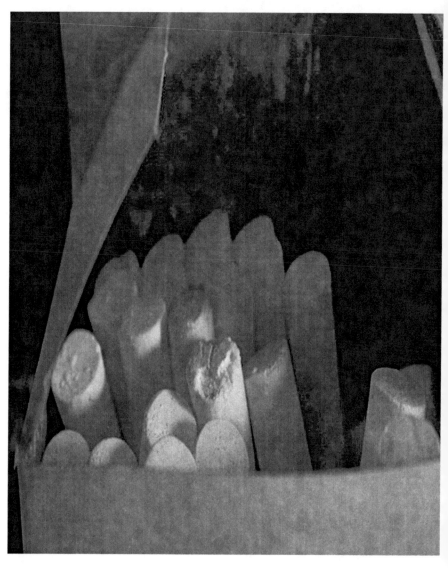

Teachers Tools
by Sakkra Paiboon

Making a Difference as a Nurse Educator
Alisa Olson

As educators, we often get so caught up in the process of teaching and providing formative feedback that we can forget the importance and the power of positive reinforcement to our students. The student-teacher dynamic is a complex paradigm that forms an important, shared relationship. This is especially true for nurses, as the profession attracts caregiver-type individuals interested in helping others. One of the major benefits of being a nurse is being able to help those who cannot help themselves, and receiving affirmation that they, as nurses, are making a difference.

I entered the nursing profession when I was in my mid-thirties. Prior to entering the field of nursing I was a secretary in a doctor's office. I wanted to become more involved with caring for patients—not just typing their reports and sending out their bills. I was fortunate to get a job as a nurse after graduation, as there was a glut of nurses in the market! I worked for a year on a surgical floor, after a three-month training fellowship and orientation. That first year was very challenging and I often left my shift in tears, only to go home and have nightmares—usually around the theme of failure to rescue my patients. I was never able to get my work completely done or do the things I wanted to do for my patients in my 8-hour shift. I felt inadequate, as if I was the worst nurse on the planet.

After that first terrible year, I had the opportunity to transfer to the ICU. I loved this change, but it proved to be the most difficult thing I have ever done. I was trying so hard to keep up with the workload and the very steep learning curve of those first few months. The fears I had of harming my patients and feelings of inadequacy were even worse in this environment. Much of the feedback I got seemed negative; it seemed like I was always doing something wrong. Somehow I made it through the orientation successfully, in spite of my fear, on a daily basis, that I would fail. Once I was on my own, my fears and feelings of inadequacy heightened, almost to the level of paranoia. I was so afraid of making a mistake and felt everyone was waiting for me to do something really horrible. It was at this point in time that a few simple words by a manager caused a major change in my life as a nurse.

My manager's words were: "You're doing a really good job." Amazing! These few words seem insignificant now as I write them, but at the time, they were a turning point in my career. I doubt my manager ever knew she had created such a profound, defining moment for me. It is these precious opportunities that we, as instructors, all need to be on the look out for in order to help our students.

Students are in a constant mode of absorbing information, learning processes and concepts. Then, somehow, they are asked to pull all this information together into a meaningful way and apply it to their practice. The instructor's task is to assist in this rapid learning process, being sure the students do not err or get off track. The hierarchy that is forged by this student-teacher relationship is a normal byproduct of the dynamic relationship, but it also has a major disadvantage. The students, unfortunately, are often addressed only when their thinking or behavior in some way needs to be corrected. All too often, three important issues are forgotten: 1) all nurses are human; 2) the most powerful facet of human beings is their emotions; and 3) if there is no regular positive reinforcement of this emotional side, humans cannot learn or perform effectively.

Now having gone the full way around the track from student to teacher, I see how important it is for us as teachers to never forget the pent-up emotions our students carry inside them as they are trying to succeed. And though we cannot always temper the negative experiences our students may be going through, we must never forget the ultimate thing that makes us humans—our feelings. Who knows which words, seemingly simple on the surface, will be the defining moment in someone's career, affirming what they are doing right and making a difference.

As I approach the end of my nurse educator program and reflect back on this experience, I realize that what I learned from it will make me a better teacher. I cannot overlook the power of positive affirmation that helps build confidence and makes students continue to strive to improve. I must forever look for those timely, teachable moments when I can make a difference!

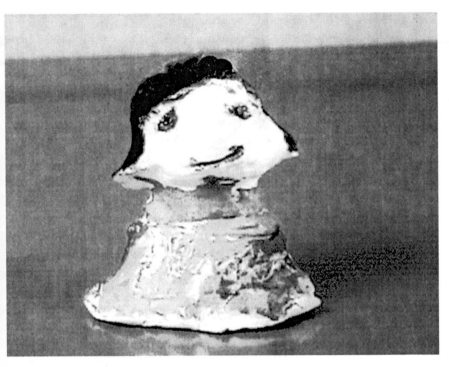

Marian in Clay
by Anonymous

My Hero
Marian Harmon

I have always enjoyed my experiences in clinical practice, working hard to care for sick patients and trying to improve the quality of life for many. Now, I look forward to my work as a nurse educator, helping future nurses to enjoy the wonderful satisfaction of nursing.

Nursing has given me the opportunity to work in highly specialized areas, such as burn and trauma and neonatal intensive care. It was important to me, at the time, to be able to "get into the trenches" and experience lifesaving procedures in order to feel that I was practicing nursing to the fullest. What could be more gratifying than bringing someone back to life?

My most recent nursing experiences have been a bit different. As the public health nurse in three schools, I have been responsible for more than 1,000 students. They range in age from pre-school to twelfth grade. The families come from all socioeconomic groups, educational levels, and ethnic backgrounds. Many families in my schools have no medical home or health insurance. One of the biggest responsibilities of my job is connecting families to services they require to take care of their health needs so they have the greatest opportunity to learn.

One very special student, Margaret, was a third grader at the elementary school. She did not have many friends her age that she played with and she often appeared sad in school. She soon became known as a "frequent flyer" to the school health clinic, coming with somatic complaints. Sometimes, she seemed to just need a moment to take a break. The family was known to have many complex social issues. Margaret often showed up at school in worn-out clothes and disheveled hair. She would always make a point to stop by the school clinic to say "Hi" or tell me a story about her weekend activities. Her little smile would reveal a mouthful of cavities and splintered teeth. Her face was scarred from a serious dog bite. I soon realized that I was one of the few people who spent some quality time with Margaret.

As the nurse in the school, I often work autonomously, but at the same time it is easy to feel out of touch and alone when it comes to making decisions about students. I was determined to work especially hard to help Margaret's mother get the health care services her child needed. This required constant communication and follow-up. Margaret needed major dental work to save her teeth and medical appointments with specialists over concerns about a gait problem that seemed to be worsening. I was overwhelmed with the needs of this one child. Her family had enough on their plate; health concerns were not a top priority at this time. I knew I would never solve all of her problems, but I really wanted to make an effort to focus on the issues that had the greatest impact on her ability to participate in school activities. Of additional concern was her poor self-esteem.

The school year marched on. Margaret was seen by a dentist and an orthopedic specialist but a lot was still in the works for her. I continued to see Margaret in the hallways and during her usual visits to the clinic. One day while I was buried in paperwork, Margaret quietly approached me at my desk. She had a little sculpture in her hands that she had made in art class. "Here," she said. I was puzzled. What was this? "Here, this is for you," she responded. "We had to make a sculpture of our hero … and I made it of you!" She beamed proudly with her black-toothed grin. I have never been so deeply touched. She made me realize why I was there and why this job was so meaningful. Just by taking the time to visit with her, listen, and try to help her get the medical treatment she needed, I had apparently made a difference to this child. It felt so good. She was really *my* little hero! To this day, I keep a picture of the sculpture on my desk to remind me not only of her, but of why I love my job.

Today, I see that look on the faces of nursing students who come to me, their new preceptor, for their pediatric rotation in school health. Margaret is there with me, as I think about how I might make a difference for these students. I know when they arrive and I introduce myself as a public health nurse here in the school, they begin to wonder, "How am I going to get a pediatric experience here … there are no PIC lines, ET tubes, IVs or coding patients; these nurses just take temperatures and hand out bandaids and ice!" On day one, I know I have my work cut out for me, but I am determined to make a difference. My goal is to provide these nursing students with learning opportunities and to connect their classroom learning to real life nursing. School health nursing has many opportunities to develop a student's expertise in pediatrics and community health. You just have to seek it out; it is never handed to you on a platter. I know I can make a difference not only with the families I serve, but also with the nursing students who come to learn. I want these students to know that being a school nurse is so much more than bandaids and ice!

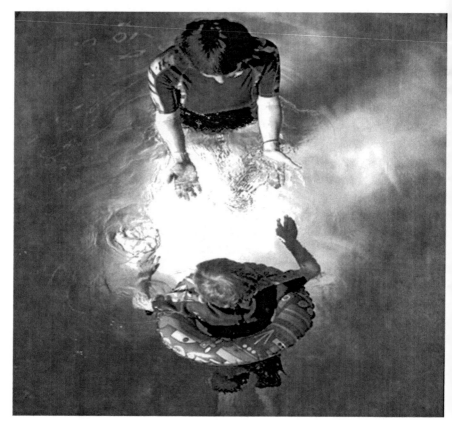

Swimmingly
by Christ Darling

Room to Grow
Shirley Pearson

When I make a difference in a patient's or their family's life, I feel part of my purpose in life is being fulfilled. Helping others is part of my spiritual being. Providing patients with kindness, safety, and assisting them with physical, emotional and spiritual care gives me a sense of meaning. Nursing is the art of caring. This philosophy extends to everyone, including students and peers.

I remember back to my days in clinical education when everything revolved around the nursing faculty. They sat upon that pedestal where everything they did, you believed was worth role modeling. The atmosphere was not one that facilitated or fostered new or creative ideas. You did it their way or you failed.

remember my first IM injection; the instructor grabbed my hand and assisted me. I felt disheartened. There was no communication from the instructor if I was doing something wrong or if she did that with all nurses on their first shot. How frustrated I was, never knowing what she was going to do to me next!

During my senior year I overheard a group of three nursing faculty discussing and laughing about a particular student's actions. My respect for those instructors diminished. I felt badly for the student whose name they mentioned. We were all working so hard and looking for guidance. That could have been any one of us. We were students who were searching for role models to help mentor us and teach us about what it means to be a nurse. I was shocked by such unprofessional behavior exhibited by the esteemed faculty I had highly respected. I knew I didn't want to be that type of nurse.

I think for any learning to take place, you have to create a safe environment. This includes respecting students as people. My mother used to say, as many other mothers have said, "treat others as you would have them treat you, and if you don't have anything nice to say, don't say anything at all." There is much to learn from these old adages.

Once a safe harbor is provided, students feel more at ease that their character will not be judged or torn down. Providing a safe environment allows the student to feel more at ease in coming to you and asking questions. If I know a student is performing a skill for the first time, we review the steps in that procedure. Depending on the comfort level of the student, he or she may only need me there for support and to catch them if they should stumble, while other students need to focus and think totally about the skill while I will talk with the patient.

Besides respect and safety, students need to know they won't be alone, that the instructor is there for them, almost like a parent. Providing clear guidelines, direction, and support are other teaching methods students need. Students, like adult learners, use stories and lessons learned to aid in their own growth. It is amazing to see the "light bulbs" go off—those "ah, ha" moments! During one of my evaluation summaries from nursing students this past year, they requested more real life stories from clinical practice. They enjoy sharing their clinical stories in post conference. Students learn as they teach one another. They are able to benefit from the clinical experiences of others.

It is important to know each student's goals and needs. Prior to the first clinical day, I have the students write out their goals, needs, and the clinical skills they would like to accomplish for the rotation. My hopes are to open the doors of communication. A goal of mine is to determine how much room the student needs to grow without feeling smothered. The difficult part, the real art of teaching, is finding that magic balance between giving them enough information to make their own discoveries without handing them everything on a silver platter. Providing students with small steps of freedom in their new practice provides them with an increasing self confidence and reassurance that they are acquiring necessary and useful skills. Sharing the moment of discovery with a student is what I find so rewarding. Being able to make a difference in the education of a nurse makes all the other trials and tribulations encountered along the way seem worthwhile.

Asking Questions
Paige Migliozzi

I have always felt nursing has been more of a "calling" than a job. I think if we truly listen to our calling, our hearts will guide us how to make a difference in our patients' lives. I always try to make eye contact with my patients and hold their hands. I feel this makes a huge difference in connecting with someone during a difficult time and letting them know we, as nurses, care and are there for them.

I feel many students will be "scared" to talk to a patient or hold their hand. I will encourage them that over time, they will begin to feel more comfortable with their patient interactions. I think the nursing home rotation is always a great place for students to begin; it allows them to start at the primary heart of nursing—communication.

I also feel many students are scared to ask questions from older nurses for fear of looking "stupid" or "unprepared". I also encourage my Operating Room fellows to acknowledge that the best thing you can do for your patients is to ask questions! If you never do a procedure, you will never know anything. Students need not to be intimidated by the older more experienced nurses; they need to take initiative to learn. The biggest difference you can make in a patient's life is to provide them with safe practice!

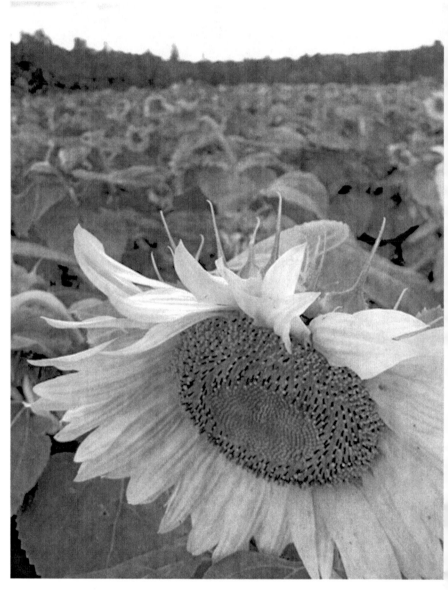

Cloudy Day in Sunflower Field
by Chris Darling

GI "Jane" as Patient Advocate

Hettie C. Mercer

This nurse's love of her specialty translates into her providing exceptional care to her patients and to her fellow staff members.

As a GI nurse with 21 years of clinical experience in a hospital Endoscopy unit, I feel an obligation to share my passion for GI nursing with students and with newly hired nurses. I often think back to how difficult it was when I transferred from a medical-surgical unit to Endoscopy 20 years ago. The orientation I received was mainly task-focused: learning the correct way of handling the different types of high-tech equipment, assist in complicated procedures, taking multiple biopsies, etc. The satisfaction of caring for patients had taken a back seat until I had mastered all the "tasks". Needless to say, the first six months were tremendously difficult and thoughts of leaving were in my mind everyday. I felt more like a technician than a nurse. Moreover, there was barely any educational literature on GI-related conditions and procedures on the unit.

My feelings of inadequacy and dissatisfaction vanished when a new head nurse was hired who encouraged me to attend educational meetings offered by the Society of Gastroenterology Nurses and Associates. Besides the educational knowledge I gained from the lectures and workshops, networking with other GI nurses gave me the boost I needed to put my heart back into my work. I started to focus on the patients again, easing their fears, providing comfort, teaching them about GI conditions, and ensuring their safety. As my confidence grew, my love for GI nursing grew as well. Knowing that you can prevent colon cancer through regular colorectal screening and removal of polyps alone makes being a GI nurse worthwhile, and educating patients and families is satisfying. Knowing that you can prevent a patient from having major surgery through endoscopic treatment of GI bleeding is another reason to love GI nursing. But the most important reason is that you directly can make a difference in the patient's experience of this perceived "unpleasant" procedure. If the patient has an unpleasant experience, it is unlikely he or she is going to return for follow up procedures; that is where nurses make a difference.

Since my orientation 20 years ago, our GI unit has grown from four employees to a staff of 35 nurses and techs. When I became the charge nurse 15 years ago, one of the first things I did was to develop a better orientation program in collaboration with the Education and Training department. There is now an educational and "hands-on" component to orientation of new nurses in conjunction with the use of preceptorship. Ongoing support and camaraderie from team members has helped new nurses to grow and become competent members of the team. I can proudly say that it is rare when one of our nurses leave. As a matter of fact, the few that did leave, retired or relocated. Yes, nurses employed in specialty units must learn the skills necessary, but in order to keep them there, they must find value in their work by putting caring for patients, family, and team members as the priority. After all, that is what nurses like doing the best. Building a culture of ongoing education and support for students and staff truly can make a difference in drawing new nurses to the profession, as well as retaining the ones we have.

A Defining Moment
Karen Livornese

The most memorable events in my career when I felt very good about making a difference were the times I had to hold my breath, put fear aside, and dive right in …

One of these incidents happened about four years ago. I was working as an evening charge nurse on a research, child psychiatry unit. A ten-year old boy was admitted to our unit for observation of child-onset schizophrenia. The family was from Vermont. They were very liberal, did not like rules, and were heavily involved in an alternative life style. Well, a family that disregards rules on a psych unit is bad news for anyone. The staff had difficulty tolerating the family, especially the father. He would get his son from the dinner table, turn him around in the same chair, and then turn on the television—even though there were other children still eating and staff was right there. Every evening he would come in and test some limit. He would wait for the staff to react and then roll his eyes, blow out of his mouth, and make a snide remark about how unintellectual the staff was. I have to say—he was by far one of my least favorite people. Every time the door buzzer would go off and I saw him on the other side of the door, I could feel my mind and body chemically react to his presence. But I was the charge nurse and was determined not to let him affect me professionally.

One evening, the father was on the unit and the usual scenario played out. Father tested a limit on the rules and the nurse needed to address the situation—nothing new. But, out of the corner of my eye, I saw the father heading, or shall I say "storming" out the door. I knew there was something wrong. The easiest thing to do was to let him go and enjoy the rest of my evening. Although I thought briefly about taking this easy way out, I knew I had to do something.

I ran to the end of the hall and met him in the threshold of the entrance to the unit, just before the door was closing. I said, "Mr. Smith—you don't look happy. What happened?" Initially, he looked completely shocked—shocked that anyone actually cared about how he was feeling. After about a 10 second silence, he told me that he didn't like the nurse working with his son; she was too harsh and she was chewing gum (Nicorrette) and it was making him angry. He just started "flooding". I told him that I understood how he felt and that actually the whole staff understood the tremendous sorrow and heartache he has everyday when he sees his son and knows that he will never have a normal life. I assured him that we did not see his son as a patient, but as an adorable kid with a sweet and quirky sense of humor who was helping us with our research.

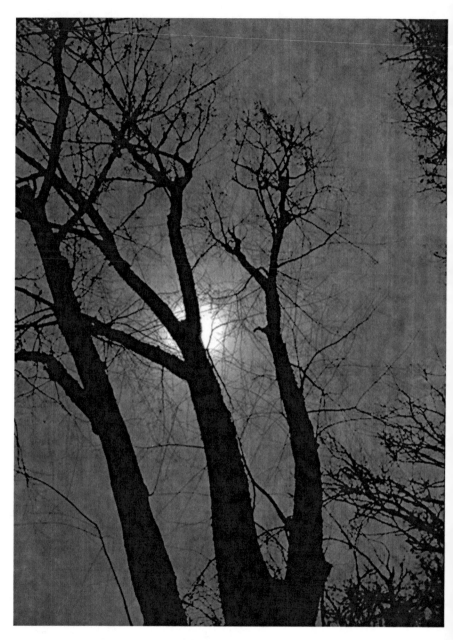

Halo Rounds the Moon
by Chris Darling

After our little chat, there was a brief smile from him. His son was with us for six additional months. His father never had a problem with the staff or the unit rules after our talk. In fact, he was quite pleasant.

This incident has stayed with me. It's because I faced one of my fears—confrontation—and went forward and dove in and addressed the problem (even when there was an easy way out). The outcome was the best possible—a content parent and a happy staff. I also learned a valuable lesson—not to assume that the patient on the unit is the only one who needs care. Yes, I know; we learned about caring for the whole family in nursing school. But, this gentleman was in his mid-thirties, in good, physical health, and gainfully employed—not "I need help" material. Unfortunately, his behaviors were so unappealing that the staff distanced themselves from him because he caused so much angst on the unit. What really needed to happen was for the staff to get closer to him. But how was I ever going to experience this success first hand if I didn't leave my introverted world of non-confrontation? People do not want to step out of their comfort zone. But I stepped out of my comfort zone and made a difference!

The feeling of this type of success is something every nursing student should feel. My guess is that they are constantly stepping out of their comfort zone, especially on their first day of clinical. But it is important to not get too comfortable or you may miss something—like I did with Mr. Smith. This is why I remember this incident very clearly. For me, it was a defining moment.

Making a Difference in a Life
Nadia Ali

To make a difference in anyone's life, one should work on qualities like genuine acceptance and empathy. I learned about these principles when I was researching learning theories and read about Carl Rogers's experiential learning. I started believing in these important qualities. First, you have to be genuine to yourself then you can be genuine to others and accept persons as who they are, not the behavior they are presenting at that moment. It is important to be empathetic and try to fit in their shoes. You have to have these qualities if you want to be effective in any relationship, whether student/teacher or patient/nurse. If you don't have these qualities, no matter what kind of technology or technique you use to try to improve students' attitudes towards learning or behavior change, you will never see the improvement.

I will share an example where I think I made a difference in patient attitude. This patient came to the ER around 10:00 am with exacerbation of COPD. He spent seven hours in the ER. He asked for his routine medication orders, emphasizing many times that he wanted the medications on time, but nobody had time to listen to his concern. He came to my unit around 5:00 pm, unhappy and still asking for his medications. The nurse on the floor was very busy and could not attend to his concern. His stress level went up and he started threatening the nurses. One of the managers talked to him but nothing helped. Finally, by 7:30 pm, he received some of his meds but he was not happy.

I came at 7:00 pm and got report that this client was very unhappy, I got a little excited because I wanted to see if I could use genuine acceptance and empathy and if it would work. I went to his room, introduced myself, confirmed his name and then reflected on his feelings. I told him: "I know you are very unhappy at this time and I agree with your frustration. We did not provide you with the care the way you wanted but I really want you to be content. How can I help you to decrease your frustration?" He started complaining again and repeated the same story. I listened patiently without passing judgment, explaining what other medication he will be receiving. He had a concern about IV Solu-Medrol because it increased his blood sugar and he received insulin. At home his sugar level was well controlled and he wanted the dose that he was taking at home. Since he had concerns with his medication, I told him I would call his physician. I paged the physician and explained the situation and concern of the patient. At first, the physician was reluctant to talk with the patient but then he agreed and listened to the same complaint. He agreed to change the medication order as the patient wanted. Later, I went to the patient's room and gave him the update and told him the medication order had been changed.

You know what he told me? "You are very kind." I saw on his face all his anger, frustration, and stress had vanished. I saw a very kind man. He slept that night peacefully without any more complaint.

If a student comes to you with all kinds of frustration, please give him the benefit of a doubt and use these principles. Who knows—maybe it will work for you too and you may get a chance to make a difference in students' lives.

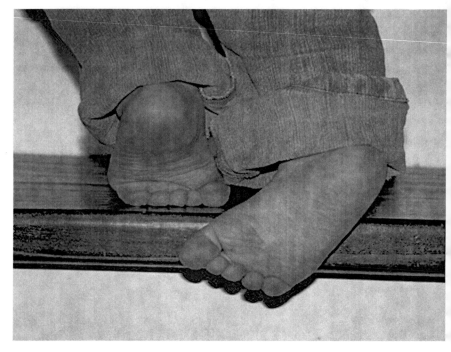

Baby Feet 3
by Nichole Manner

Little "Feats" of Wonder
Nagaina Simmons

A Neonatal Intensive Care Nurse gives her all to her patients and their families.
Being a neonatal intensive care nurse is definitely my calling. I couldn't imagine
working with any other patient population. Babies are resilient little beings and
in my experience, most get better and go home with their parents and families. I
become attached to some babies more than others. In a lot of these cases, it's
because of the relationship that I have with the parents. When you're a NICU
nurse, you're not only focusing on caring for the baby, but you must also remember to care for and educate the parent(s); after all, once the baby gets better, they
are the ones that must care for the infant from there on out. Developing a positive relationship with the parents is critical in neonatal nursing care.

I remember one set of parents that I developed a really good relationship with.
Their first son, Baby M., was born around 28 weeks and stayed in the NICU for
several months. I had the opportunity to care for him a lot during the course of

the stay. At that time, I was getting more comfortable in my role as a neonatal nurse, so I spent a lot of time answering questions and educating these parents about their preemie. They knew me by name and were always glad to see me even if I wasn't caring for their son. Eventually, Baby M. got healthy enough, and big enough, to go home. Unfortunately, I wasn't able to be there when he was discharged (I was on vacation). But before I left, the parents told me how thankful they were for the care that I gave their son and for the attention that I gave them. That's when I knew that I was exactly where I was supposed to be, where I needed to be.

The story doesn't end there. About three years later, the same parents had another son, Baby T., who was born around 34 weeks and came to the NICU. His stay was much shorter than that of his brother. I remember being so excited to see the parents again, hoping that they would remember me. And you know what? They did! I really didn't take care of him as much as I did his brother, but I would always go and talk with the parents whenever they came in to visit. About a week later, after he was discharged, I was working the night shift when the father called to say that he was in the ER with Baby T., who was having trouble breathing. The father sounded very distressed and worried, so immediately the neonatologist and I walked down to the ER. When we got there, I could see how elated the father was to see us. He expressed that he was very frustrated with the ER staff and didn't feel like they "knew what they were doing". The neonatologist immediately assessed Baby T., drew blood, and instructed me to start an IV. After about 30 minutes, the results came back that he had respiratory syncytial virus (RSV). He was to be transferred to another facility for care. Just before they left, the father expressed how grateful he was that we came down to take care of his son. I remember him saying to me: "I'm so glad that you were working tonight." That has stayed with me ever since.

As I grow as a clinician, I am starting to realize how much of a difference I make for my patients and their families. I am their caregiver, teacher, counselor, and advocate. If I want to make a difference for my future students, I must also take on these roles. First, as their teacher, it is my responsibility to equip them with the knowledge and skills they will need to become excellent clinicians. Being a caregiver and counselor is almost second nature to us as nurses. I believe it's important to remember that students are not just students. They have families, beliefs, and past experiences; in other words, other things besides school are an important part of their lives and affect them as individuals. It is important to be flexible and to remember that they may need you to be available to them when issues or problems arise. Being an advocate to my students is just as important as it is with my patients. This role arises particularly in the clinical part of nursing academia, where I may have to stand up for my students if issues arise with staff or patients. I want to listen, understand, encourage, and support my students. To put it best, I want to "be available" to meet their needs.

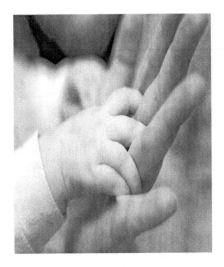

Hands
By Alp Timurnan Cevik

Making a Difference in a Journey
Fleur D. May

It has always been my goal to give the most caring and competent care I can give to my mother/baby patients. Taking the time to make a difference in their postpartum stay goes a long way in improving the patients' perceptions of their care, which directly affects positive patient outcomes. While it is important to assess the learning needs of patients, it is equally important to match curriculum and teaching styles with the learning needs of new hires and nursing students.

Two years ago, I had the opportunity to precept a George Mason student in her senior year, and with her assistance, to streamline a teaching/learning strategy. Using the George Mason Preceptor Workbook and the student's syllabus as a framework, a six week schedule of objectives was agreed upon. A contract was worked out to clarify student and preceptor responsibilities, and a timeline for accomplishing objectives was established.

Four weeks into the clinical rotation, the student was exhibiting professional behaviors and was completing assessments and patient care on three mother/baby pairs, with the appropriate level of competence and autonomy as outlined in the George Mason syllabus. It was about this time that a patient came into our lives that afforded an opportunity for the student to manage a patient with rapidly changing acuity ...

Together we admitted a patient who was two hours postpartum from an emergency Cesarean section surgery. The mom was stable on admission, and we received a report from the labor and delivery nurse that was unremarkable for history. The patient's husband and mother were at the bedside. The student was familiar with the standard of care for a C-Section patient. After obtaining the first set of vital signs, the student made notes as I relayed information about my hands-on assessment. The patient had been with us one hour when the second assessment was due.

As we entered the patient's room for the second assessment, there was a noticeable difference. Our patient was clammy and pale, had a normal respiration rate and temperature, but had an increased heart rate (HR 140). The blood pressure was 100/60. After making a preliminary assessment and ruling out a postpartum hemorrhage, a nasal cannula with 3 liters of oxygen was placed on the patient. I asked the student to gather supplies for starting an IV. Then I started making phone calls: first to the doctor, and then to my charge nurse. I had a feeling I was looking at either a postpartum hemorrhage, or possible pulmonary embolism. I remained at the bedside and waited for the obstetrician to arrive.

Within minutes, the doctor was at the bedside evaluating the situation, ordering labs and x-rays. At one point, we had the nurse manager, the charge nurse, the doctor, and a nurse's aide in the room with us, offering assistance. Everyone was professional, attentive, and reassuring to both the patient and to her husband and mother. The student was also comforting to the family. The patient was eventually transferred to the Intensive Care Unit with a falling blood pressure and tachycardia.

While we were involved with our acute patient, the charge nurse assumed responsibility for the other two mother/baby pairs assigned to us. After documenting the transfer, a short debrief was made. The student recalled how smoothly the collaboration and communication went, and how following the nursing process assisted the doctor in making a diagnosis and treatment plan. This made the student feel secure that in a similar situation, her colleagues would support her. I made sure I commended her on her professionalism and her efforts to comfort the family.

Although we had this patient a short time, I believe we made a difference to the patient and her family, in keeping them updated and informed, while making sure every resource was followed up that related to providing her with safe care. The patient's family sought us out after the patient was transferred to thank us for supporting them and keeping them informed. Again, this was a unique opportunity to mentor a student through a stressful situation, watch her grow as a nurse, and make a difference in her journey as a future nurse.

Mentoring Clinical Nurse Educators of the Future

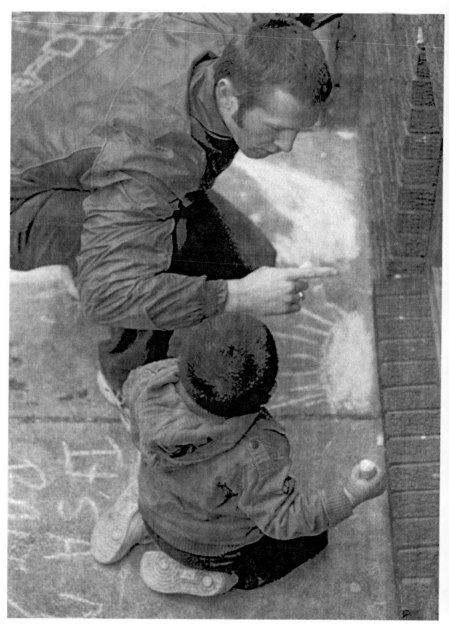

The Lesson
by Ed Hall

Even Teachers Need A Little Guidance Now and Then

Amy O'Neill

I will never forget that phone call. I was lazing on my couch, sprawling in the easness of a day off and recovering from a crazy day on the unit the day before. I had bounced from delivery to delivery, and I had helped my orientee, Virginia, understand the importance of palpating contractions, even when the patient had an intrauterine pressure catheter. I was exhausted but satisfied. Then, the phone rang.

It was Joanne, the new hire coordinator, and she greeted me with a cheery spout of words that would ill prepare me for the news she was bearing. I was still wondering what the point of her calling was, when Joanne let the guillotine fall. "So Amy, I was talking with Virginia yesterday, about how her orientation is going. She says that things are going really well, she feels very confident in her skills and she feels comfortable in patient care situations. So that's great." "Yeah, that is great," I echoed, feeling somewhat wary about where this was going. Joanne plowed on. "Dolores took her on for the day, when you were sick, and she expressed that Dolores was a really good fit as preceptor for her. In fact, she suggested that, maybe she could spend more time with Dolores. Maybe you and Dolores could share her. Now, let me make this clear: Virginia expressed that she felt you were an excellent preceptor, but she just felt that she and Dolores were a better fit."

I was devastated. In fact, as I struggled to collect Joanne's words, and as the weight of their meaning smashed into my brain, I fell apart. I started sobbing on the phone to Joanne. I had failed. I was a horrible preceptor. I had tried so hard, put myself out there with no training and no guidance, to be the best preceptor I could be. I had experimented with novel, interactive, hands-on lessons, photocopied relevant articles, and pushed Virginia just out of her range of comfort, into such frustration that I had left her no choice but to abandon me. I had failed, on my very first try.

I struggled the rest of that week. I would see Virginia in the hallways, be afraid to look her in the eye, and fear the eyes of all the other nurses. Did they know? Had Virginia told them horrible things about me? As the week went on, sure enough, people started noticing that Virginia was not orienting with me. I had to come up with answers, some politically correct, positive-sounding answers that I never actually believed. For that week, I would have to take Virginia back, and I would have to remain professional in behavior; inside I could barely contain my sadness and anger. I felt betrayed. The one girl whom I had embraced as the first of many students, had demolished my hopes of becoming a teacher of nursing.

Where had I gone wrong? I reviewed the last two months, examined our interactions, and began to see the cracks. I had been overly demanding. I had pushed Virginia too hard. I had tried new ways of teaching, but they were not what she had needed. Crumbled and despairing, I went to the one person I knew who could help me: Barb. Barb was like me, fast-forwarded 30 years. Barb was dreaming of a career in nursing education, and she was in a master's program. She had been a labor and delivery nurse for thirty years, and she had a passion for teaching new hires. I considered Barb my mother figure on the unit, the gentle embrace I could go to for a listening ear, a guiding hand, and a warm hug. Barb was my mentor.

I took Barb aside on the unit during a particularly quiet day. I told her everything: the call, the devastation, the fallout. She took me into an empty labor room, and she hugged me. She looked into my eyes, and she said something that would stay with me for years to come: "Amy, you know, even though you're a teacher, you still have to learn how to teach." I was startled, and I did not entirely understand what she meant. She went on: "Nobody knows how to teach when they first begin. This time did not work out; you probably did push Virginia too hard. You know, you always have to keep in mind your student when you are teaching. You have to adjust your methods to the person. This was your first time teaching. Do not get depressed about it. Learn from it. You'll do better next time."

I looked at her, questioning. "Maybe there shouldn't be a next time. Maybe I'm just not cut out for this."

Barb smiled. "Of course you are. You cannot let this one time get you down. You are going to be a great teacher some day. Get through this experience, and learn from it."

"But, what about the other nurses? I mean, I know they know what happened. I just feel so stupid!"

"Don't worry about it!" Barb assured me. "They may know, but they don't really care. Don't let it get to you." With a hug, Barb sent me off, shaken but stirred on to a new start. I absorbed all of what had just happened, and I processed what it all meant to me.

Suddenly, I felt rejuvenated—and free. I did not have to be the Perfect Teacher. I could make mistakes. Moreover, I could make those mistakes in front of everyone, and it would still be okay. They would forget, but I would carry with

ne valuable lessons for the future. I realized how much I needed Barb, my men-
or, how I could not be confident and strong all the time, and how teachers need
a little guidance every now and then. I would finish orienting Virginia and many
other students in the future, but I would not have to do it alone. After all, teachers need each other.

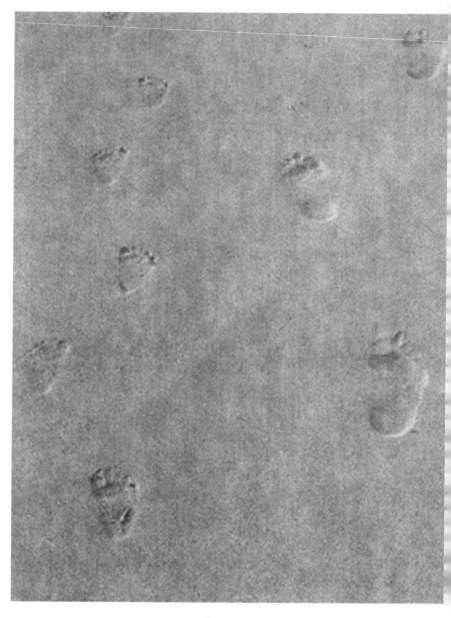

Footsteps
by Anonymous

A Thousand Little Steps
Karen Backo

I have always enjoyed the education process, be it as a student or the one imparting information. When I graduated in 1996 with my baccalaureate degree in nursing from Loma Linda University in Southern California, my graduating class voted me "Most Likely to Teach at Loma Linda". As an already practicing RN, I knew the value of continuing education. Practicing in a teaching institution provided plenty of opportunities to educate new nurses, patients, and the very new doctors beginning their residency. The educators at Loma Linda had prepared a strong foundation for my journey to academe. And, although at the time I remember wondering "what on earth my fellow students saw in me", as I reflect on my journey to 2008, the skills of an educator have indeed emerged. As I traveled on this path, I have had both the opportunity to mentor and be mentored. What I have most appreciated, are the individuals who have believed in my abilities as an educator and afforded me the opportunities to educate in both the clinical and classroom setting. I have the utmost appreciation for my graduate professors who have encouraged, undergirded, and assisted in the development of my teaching skills. Some of them have had to observe my "skills" numerous times and have been ever so patient and gracious with their time and talent. I hope that it is gratifying for them to know that their legacy will continue on in the work of their students. As I reflect on my thousand little steps toward becoming a nurse educator, what is clear is the immense challenge of the educating profession and the profound responsibility we have toward tomorrow's nurses and the quality of health care that they will provide.

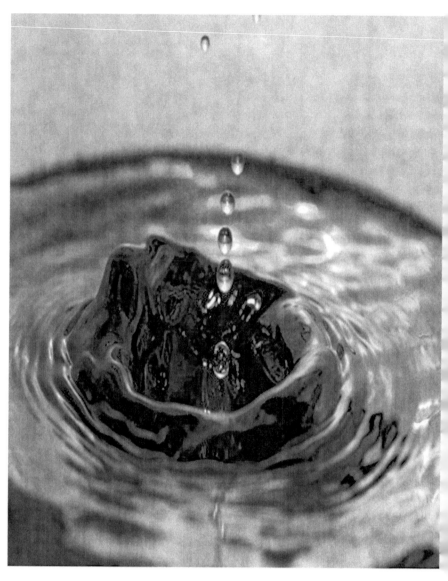

Water Droplets
By Son Nguyen

Each Individual is Unique
Deirdre Dorsey

A few years ago, new hire nurses were assigned to a clinical nurse mentor for orientation which was structured to be accomplished in a year, producing a fully functioning clinic nurse. One of the new hires was an older nurse returning to patient care after several years of working in risk management. She was enthusiastic, pleasant, and a team player. The challenges arose when the orientation program schedule exceeded her learning pace. Attending the didactic lecture sessions, applying the nursing clinical skills, and managing patient charts was posing difficulty and frustration for her. In addition, administering immunizations to infants and small children seemed to be a particular obstacle causing anxiety.

The clinical nurse mentor took steps to help the new nurse through meetings to identify each concern and problem; then they jointly worked on each issue. The mentor's additional time with one-on-one clinical instruction, extra appropriate materials/videos, and encouragement allowed this new hire to successfully complete the orientation program. Recognizing that each individual is unique and that learning occurs differently for some were key factors to restructuring and extending her orientation. She became a valuable clinic team member and enjoyed her new experiences in patient care.

As I reflect on this story, the role of a mentor for a novice clinical nurse educator becomes more defined. My ideas of what I may need from a mentor include: a) an open and honest relationship; b) an opportunity to observe, assist, and participate in teaching; c) introduction to new thoughts, skills, and techniques; d) guidance with teaching assignments; e) working with a dedicated preceptor; f) experiencing a network of novice to expert nurse educators; g) flexibility with assignments and class schedules; and h) learning new nursing skills/tools to be quite successful in this journey.

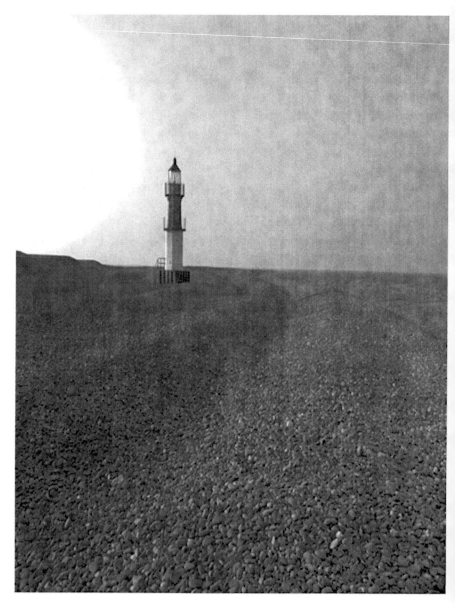

Point of Ayre Lighthouse
by Tony Hisgett

Positive Attitude
Emily Sperlazza

I had the opportunity to present information about simulation at a community college gathering for the state. I went with several faculty members from my college and felt very supported by them. After I did my presentation, the faculty members gave me a lot of encouragement and praise. I feel that most of the faculty at my college mentor me—they seem at ease with that role and provide me with very good models of how to mentor. I feel valued and supported, and know that they are experienced and knowledgeable and will help me any way they can.

I think that mentors need to approach students with a positive attitude and be strength-based, though that doesn't mean pretending everything is wonderful if it isn't. It's also important to be honest with students in a way that is sensitive to the situation and their feelings.

Also, I think being non-judgmental is a critical trait for mentors. You need to encourage students to ask questions and be honest about their capabilities and areas for growth. If you are judgmental, you will shut students down and they may get into trouble more easily.

It's also helpful when mentors are good listeners. If you listen well to students, you will be much more aware of what their needs are and how to support them. Mentors need to individualize their approach to their students and recognize each student's needs and strengths.

I think it's also important that mentors not micro-manage their students. Students need to understand what's expected of them, and then be allowed to fulfill those expectations without an instructor watching every move they make. Mentors, however, need to be readily available to students, not only in terms of a physical presence, but also in terms of being a resource to the students.

When I think of those people in my life who have been mentors to me, I also see intelligence and integrity as important traits. Respecting what the mentor has to say is kind of an essential starting point. If a student doesn't have an interest in the mentor to begin with, then none of the rest matters. Basically, good mentoring means being able to *connect* with students, so that skills such as good listening and being strength-based will facilitate those "connections." Also, good mentors should *show the way* in terms of how they negotiate the role you are trying to adopt, so skills such as integrity and intelligence will help in creating paths for students.

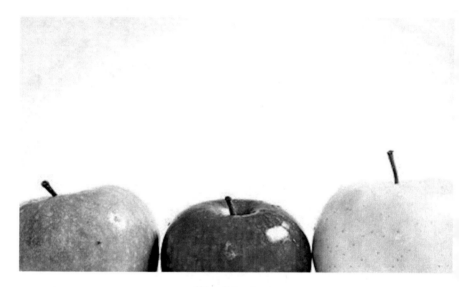

Shiny Shiny Apples
by Venysia Kurniawan

Wanted: Mentors!
Comfort Avovabey

As a novice beginning a new profession, it is always important to reeducate myself about rules and how things are done in a particular setting. Learning to be a clinical educator can be very challenging to new members because it involves moving from what you know to what you do not know. Therefore, the need for guidance from experienced or senior members is important to the learning process.

New clinical educators could seek out mentors who have similar beliefs and philosophies like themselves to help coach and guide them through the transition. In order to be successful, the new faculty member needs a mentor who has characteristics that include patience, understanding, and willingness to share knowledge, expertise, and professional experiences; to be available to give tips and tricks of the trade, as well as providing strategies for success.

Mentoring ideas should include: motivation to enrich the passion of teaching, how to interact with students and reaching out to everyone, how to create a stimulating and a good learning environment for teaching, and how to evaluate student progress.

These are among many ways that can help new members succeed in their role transition. I look forward to doing that!

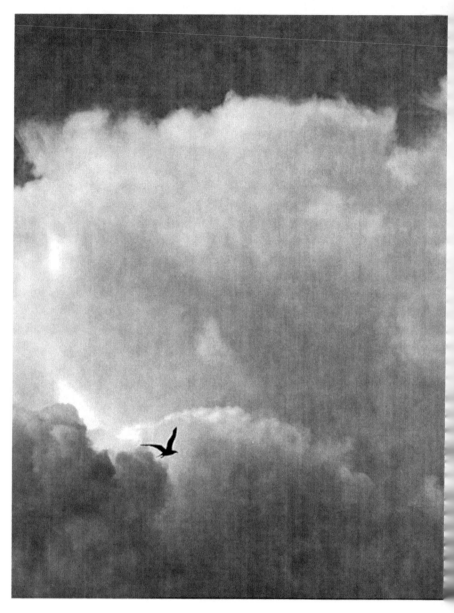

Soaring
by Matt Lyons

A Love of Nursing and a Passion to Teach
Megan M. Davis

Throughout our lives, we encounter people who inspire us and shape who we become. This story is a wonderful example of encouraging young people to consider a career in nursing ...

My nursing career began in 1966 when I was a 12 year old volunteer at West Jersey Hospital in Camden, New Jersey. At this young age, I worked 500 hours in the Central Supply Room (CSR). It was here that I was fortunate to meet my first clinical nursing mentor. The CSR was manned by one nursing supervisor (my mentor) and her band of processing experts. My job was to deliver sterile equipment to the patient floors. It was a simple job and I had limited patient contact. That was fine; I needed to learn the basics of medical equipment. However, my mentor saw in me a person who wanted to learn. Because of her generosity, I was allowed to participate in the sterile processing of needles, gloves, and sterile trays! (This was long before plastic and disposal items came to hospitals.) My mentor allowed me to grow. She also taught me to respect everyone in the room—they all had a job to do. She led by example and worked along side her people whenever necessary. I wanted to be just like her.

Much later, in 1975, I became an O.R. orderly for a children's hospital in Philadelphia. My head nurse, Jackie, became my nursing mentor. Again, Jackie saw that I wanted to do more than move patients about in the hospital. Jackie allowed me to learn to scrub. She paired me with another nurse and I got to practice handing instruments for simple surgeries. Jackie allowed me to explore surgical nursing.

These two nurses helped me identify what I, as a clinical nurse educator, need in a mentor. First there must be a love of nursing and then there must be a passion to teach. A good mentor is a person capable of great generosity. She must be willing to spend time to help others. It takes time to explain why you do what you do. A mentor needs to be willing to take a student, assess her needs, offer suggestions and opportunities, and then let her protégé go.

Mentoring to Uncover Possibilities
Sarah Mossburg

Recently I took on the task of heading up an ad hoc subcommittee of our practice council. Our Clinical Nurse Educator had mentioned multiple times that the catheter-acquired urinary tract infection rate in the hospital was significantly elevated. I enjoy quality issues and saw this as an opportunity to take on a new challenge.

I volunteered for the role to lead inquiry into this problem and pulled together the committee. The committee looked at the factors that were causing our elevated infection rate. We decided to implement a number of process improvements, one of which was to create a one-page educational flyer about urinary tract infections for the nursing staff. As head of the committee, I had done most of the background work and volunteered to create the flyer. I spent a lot of time working on it.

I got a tremendous amount of help from a coworker who I consider to be a mentor. She has a post-masters certificate in education, and has worked as an educator in the past. She helped me refine the flyer so that it would have the most impact on the educational areas that we had identified as the most crucial to decreasing our infection rate. The next step was to determine how we should roll out the educational flyer. Having never implemented a hospital-wide education campaign, I was not sure how to do it. I had already started planning an appropriate strategy but needed assistance from someone experienced who could help me refine that plan with ideas that have worked in the past. This example highlights what a mentor does; she provides helpful feedback and facilitates the learning process. My mentor doesn't tell me how to do it, she asks me what thoughts and ideas I have and then helps guide me to uncover hidden opportunities or pitfalls.

Meeting the Challenges of Nursing Education
Shirley Pearson

Education, networking, and mentoring provide the knowledge and support nurse educators need to light their way as they provide exemplary education for students, as well as working nurses.

Every new career or adventure carries with it uncertainties and unfamiliar territory. A new nursing career can be overwhelming. Having a mentor can assist you in your journey to find your way. Hopefully, like Florence Nightingale carrying her torch, your mentor will help guide your trail and provide light in the right direction.

A clinical nurse educator's duties and responsibilities are very different from a staff nurse working on a unit at the hospital. To be a successful clinical nurse educator, you must possess two knowledge bases and skill sets. You must already be advanced in your nursing practice but also have knowledge about how to teach. There are some similar aspects between the two settings, such as safety and prioritization issues. But not everyone possesses great teaching abilities.

In most acute care facilities each unit has a variety of checklists and competencies that must be completed within a specific timeframe. Job descriptions are used as a basis for competencies and evaluations of the nursing staff. Many nursing administrative or desk jobs do not have specific orientation guidelines. Educational roles are as important as clinical jobs but less attention is paid to this aspect of nursing. It surprises me that educators, with their love of detail, do not have a formal orientation to become clinical nurse educators. Educators are constantly evaluating performance and suggesting improvements but this focus does not seem to have been emphasized in clinical education.

My first experience as a clinical educator was many years ago. My qualifications for this job were clinical experience and a willingness to work with students. There was no formal education or orientation offered for my new responsibilities. Not knowing what I should know about clinical education was a bit like playing 'Pin-the-Tail on the Donkey"! I realize now that I didn't know enough to ask meaningful questions. I was in my own world. The nursing school provided me with a copy of course objectives, the student textbook was available, and a copy of the labs the students had completed, but there was so much I didn't know!

I remember being so excited about beginning my new role in clinical teaching; I wanted to share everything I knew. These students were also enthusiastic about being in the clinical setting. They were like little sponges absorbing as much as they could, or at least most of the students were like this. It is mentally challenging and exhausting trying to find ways to engage other students who do not seem interested in learning. Now I realize my teaching style may have been the problem. Without knowledge from my recent coursework, I would not be able to figure this out. Had I known then what I know now, I might have possibly stayed in that teaching arena.

What I understand now is that I need what we provide to our new orientees today in the acute care setting. For the most part, there are guidelines and timelines, very much like a course syllabus. It is important to have a list of skill and didactic information the students have covered and will cover in the weeks during clinical. Organizational tools and record keeping ideas would have been welcomed. A shadowing experience may be helpful for new clinical educators. A workshop such as the Nurse Educator Academy that covers specific topics would have been a dream come true. I didn't realize how much I didn't know about what I was doing until I'd been in the role for several years.

The sharing of information is a wonderful concept if there are educators willing to do so. Computer access presents the opportunity to share ideas and information more readily. When I first started as a nurse educator, computers were not yet introduced and everything was done by hand or a typewriter. Now there is no excuse for not sharing important information!

Another essential need for success in your new role as clinical educator includes support from staff and administration. There needs to be someone I can talk with when questions arise about polices or problem students. I also want to feel welcome where I work. I want to feel comfortable about sharing ideas. Having your opinions valued and trusted is important to being a professional. To facilitate this, it is important to have a shared expectation of goals and objectives with the staff and administration, coupled with adequate feedback to assess progress toward the shared goals.

Being a nurse mentor is a unique position. You help guide and mold an inexperienced nurse into a competent team member. Many different skills and abilities are required. One has to be a good nurse as well as a good teacher to be successful. This takes clinical experience and the guidance of an educator. It is not a role that just any clinical nurse can fill unless they possess mentoring skills and have the desire to teach. But it is a role that can be very satisfying!

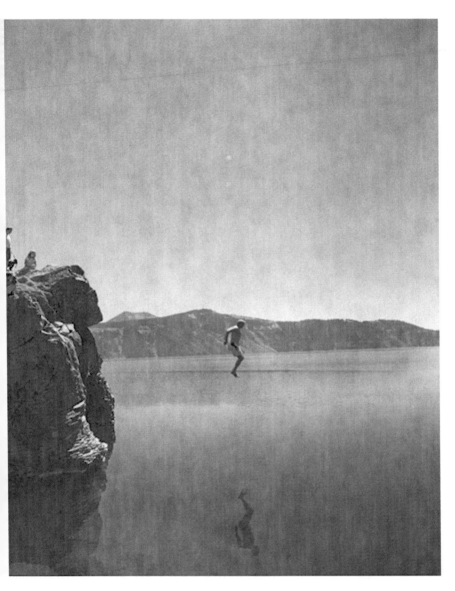

Crater Lake Mirror
by Powderruns

978-0-595-4478
0-595-44781-3

Printed in the United States
119645LV00003B/412-579/P

9 780595 447817